Vascular Dementi

Caregiver's Handl

Providing Compassionate Care for Loved Ones

Patty Boma

Copyright @2025

TABLE OF CONTENT

CHAPTER 1 4

   INTRODUCTION: THE ROLE OF THE CAREGIVER 4

CHAPTER 2 16

   COMPREHENDING VASCULAR DEMENTIA 16

CHAPTER 3 34

   DIAGNOSIS AND HEALTH CARE 34

CHAPTER 4 56

   DAILY NURTURING AND SYMPTOM MANAGEMENT 56

CHAPTER 5 79

CRAFTING A SANCTUARY OF
SAFETY AND SUPPORT 79

CHAPTER 6 100

EMOTIONAL AND MENTAL
HEALTH 100

CHAPTER 7 122

CONSIDERATIONS OF LEGAL
AND FINANCIAL NATURE...122

CHAPTER 8 140

PLANNING AHEAD FOR CARE
......................................140

CHAPTER 1

INTRODUCTION: THE ROLE OF THE CAREGIVER

The experience of caring for a cherished individual diagnosed with vascular dementia unfolds as a path marked by trials, sorrows, and instances of deep emotional bonding. This handbook serves as a guiding companion for you, the caregiver, as you journey through this intricate and frequently daunting landscape. The intention is to equip you with practical tools, offer compassionate guidance, and foster a deeper comprehension of the essence of caring for an individual with vascular dementia.

Vascular dementia stands as the second most prevalent form of dementia, following closely behind Alzheimer's disease. The condition arises from factors that obstruct the flow of blood to the brain, resulting in cognitive impairments and a deterioration in daily functioning. The path of caring for an individual with vascular dementia unfolds in a distinctive manner, marked by a specific array of symptoms, a particular progression, and unique caregiving requirements.

In the tapestry of life, your presence as a caregiver weaves a thread of profound significance for your cherished one. Your duties extend beyond mere physical care; they encompass the vital realms of emotional and psychological well-being as well. This duty may present itself as both a source of fulfillment and a formidable challenge. One must understand that caregiving resembles a marathon rather than a mere sprint. It demands a steadfast spirit, unwavering determination, and a strong network of support.

This volume seeks to equip you with the insights and tools necessary to offer the utmost care for your cherished one, all while ensuring that you also attend to your own well-being. Frequently, those who care for others overlook their own needs, resulting in exhaustion, stress, and emotional depletion. Our aim is to guide you away from such challenges by providing you with strategies for self-care and stress management, along with insights on how to seek support within your community.

In the pages that follow, we shall delve into the intricate facets of vascular dementia and the art of caregiving. From grasping the intricacies of the disease to orchestrating daily care rituals, from maneuvering through the labyrinth of the healthcare system to envisioning what lies ahead, we shall explore all the vital subjects that will aid you on this path.

The Significance of Grasping Vascular Dementia

Understanding is a formidable force. As you delve deeper into the intricacies of vascular dementia, you will find yourself better prepared to navigate the myriad challenges that lie ahead. In the opening chapters, we shall explore the essence of vascular dementia, examining its origins, manifestations, and the journey of its progression. Grasping these essential elements will lay a robust groundwork for the development of your caregiving strategies.

It is crucial to understand that vascular dementia may present itself in unique ways for each person. The manifestations of the ailment may differ, and its progression can unfold at varying paces. By delving into the prevalent patterns and possible complications, one can cultivate a sense of preparedness and proactivity in the art of caregiving.

Establishing a Network of Support

Caregiving ought to be a journey shared, never a solitary endeavor. Establishing a robust support system is essential for the well-being of both yourself and those dear to you. This volume serves as a compass, leading you to discover and forge connections with invaluable resources, encompassing healthcare professionals, support groups, and community services. The significance of engaging family and friends in the caregiving journey will also be explored.

Striking a harmonious equilibrium between the act of nurturing others and the pursuit of one's own support can prove to be a formidable challenge, yet it remains an essential endeavor. Keep in mind that seeking assistance is not indicative of frailty; rather, it reflects a profound strength and a wise perspective. Harnessing the resources at your disposal can profoundly impact both the quality of care you offer and the strength of your emotional resilience.

Embracing the Art of Self-Care

In the role of a caregiver, one must acknowledge the vital significance of self-care and the necessity of seeking support when the need arises. The burdens of caregiving can weigh heavily on one's body, heart, and mind, frequently resulting in a state of exhaustion if not navigated with care. This handbook underscores the importance of placing your well-being at the forefront, inviting you to delve into an array of strategies for self-care, stress management, and the pursuit of support from friends, family, and professional resources. It is essential to recognize that one cannot give from a vessel that is devoid of substance; nurturing oneself is not merely an indulgence, but a fundamental requirement to offer the utmost care to those we cherish.

The intent behind this handbook

"Vascular Dementia: A Caregiver's Handbook" serves as a practical and accessible guide, providing valuable insights, strategies, and support for caregivers navigating each phase of their journey. This volume is meticulously crafted to explore the myriad dimensions of caregiving, encompassing the comprehension of the medical intricacies of vascular dementia, the orchestration of daily care practices, the establishment of a secure and nurturing atmosphere, and the navigation of the emotional and legal complexities that may emerge.

CHAPTER 2
COMPREHENDING VASCULAR DEMENTIA

Vascular dementia stands as a complex and multifaceted condition, impacting millions of individuals across the globe. To provide effective and compassionate care, it is essential for a caregiver to gain a comprehensive understanding of this condition. This chapter endeavors to present a comprehensive exploration of vascular dementia, encompassing its definition, underlying causes, associated risk factors, and the symptoms that characterize this condition.

Definition and Overview

Vascular dementia emerges as a form of cognitive decline, stemming from diminished blood circulation to the brain, ultimately leading to the impairment of its cells. In contrast to other types of dementia, including Alzheimer's disease, vascular dementia is intricately linked to issues concerning the blood vessels within the brain. This form of dementia ranks as the second most prevalent, representing roughly 10-20% of all dementia occurrences. The condition may emerge abruptly in the wake of a stroke or unfold slowly as a consequence of persistent ailments that compromise the brain's blood flow.

The Underlying Causes and Contributing Risk Factors

Grasping the underlying causes and risk factors of vascular dementia is essential for effective prevention and management. Vascular dementia primarily arises from diminished blood flow to the brain, a phenomenon that may stem from various underlying conditions:

- A stroke, often referred to as a cerebrovascular accident (CVA), transpires when a blood vessel within the brain becomes obstructed by a clot, leading to an ischemic stroke, or when it ruptures, resulting in a hemorrhagic stroke. The interruption of blood flow may result in brain injury, ultimately giving rise to vascular dementia.

- Transient Ischemic Attacks, commonly known as "mini-strokes," represent fleeting episodes characterized by a temporary reduction in blood flow to the brain. While they may not inflict lasting harm, recurrent TIAs can elevate the likelihood of progressing toward vascular dementia.

- Small Vessel Disease: This ailment encompasses the deterioration of the minute blood vessels within the brain, resulting in diminished blood circulation and a slow, progressive decline in cognitive function. It frequently finds its connection with elevated blood pressure and diabetes.

- Atherosclerosis is characterized by the accumulation of fatty deposits, known as plaques, within the arteries. This condition can lead to the narrowing or obstruction of blood vessels, thereby diminishing blood flow to the brain and heightening the risk of vascular dementia.

A multitude of risk factors may heighten the chances of one developing vascular dementia. Among these risk factors, some can be altered, while others remain immutable:

- As the years accumulate, so too does the risk of vascular dementia, notably intensifying after one reaches the age of 65.

- In the realm of vascular dementia, it is observed that men tend to face a greater risk than their female counterparts.

- The lineage of one's family holds significant weight; a history marked by stroke or vascular dementia may elevate the chances of encountering such conditions oneself.

- High Blood Pressure: Hypertension stands as a formidable risk factor, casting a long shadow over the potential for both stroke and vascular dementia.

- Diabetes, when left poorly managed, has the potential to inflict harm upon the blood vessels, thereby elevating the risk of developing vascular dementia.

- The act of smoking, particularly the use of tobacco, may play a significant role in the development of atherosclerosis and various other vascular complications.

- High Cholesterol: The presence of elevated cholesterol levels may result in the accumulation of plaque within the arteries.

- Heart disease manifests in various forms, with conditions like atrial fibrillation and heart attacks serving as harbingers of greater peril. These ailments not only threaten the heart but also elevate the risk of stroke and vascular dementia, weaving a complex tapestry of health challenges.

Symptoms and Phases

The manifestations of vascular dementia can differ significantly, influenced by the degree and specific areas of brain impairment. Nevertheless, certain prevalent cognitive and behavioral symptoms warrant the attention of caregivers:

Cognitive Symptoms:

- Challenges with memory, especially the loss of short-term recall

- Challenges in the realms of planning, organization, and problem-solving
- Struggles with language manifest in the challenge of selecting the appropriate words or keeping pace with the flow of conversations.
- The faculties of judgment and decision-making are compromised.

Behavioral symptoms:

- Shifts in emotional states, including feelings of

despair, unease, or indifference
- Transformations in character, marked by heightened irritability or aggression
- Visions or false beliefs
- Challenges in engaging with others and a retreat from various pursuits

Vascular dementia is frequently categorized into stages, each reflecting the severity of the symptoms experienced.

- In the initial phase, one may encounter gentle

shifts in cognitive abilities, changes that remain understated and do not markedly disrupt the rhythms of daily life. One might experience subtle lapses in memory, struggle with intricate tasks, and encounter moments of bewilderment.

- Moderate Stage: With the advancement of the condition, the cognitive and behavioral symptoms emerge with greater intensity. Some individuals may find themselves grappling with the simplest of daily tasks, facing profound lapses in memory, and displaying notable shifts in their mood and behavior.

- Severe Stage: In the later phases of vascular dementia, individuals find themselves in need of considerable support for their everyday tasks. The shadows of memory loom large, casting a pall over the once-vibrant tapestry of communication, rendering it a struggle fraught with challenges. Among the behavioral manifestations, one might observe agitation, aggression, and even the unsettling experience of hallucinations.

Grasping the symptoms and stages of vascular dementia is crucial for caregivers, for it paves the way for timely intervention and thoughtful care planning. In acknowledging the subtle signs of vascular dementia, caregivers are empowered to pursue medical evaluation and support, thereby securing the finest care for their cherished ones.

In the forthcoming chapters, we shall embark on a profound exploration of the practical dimensions of caregiving. This journey will encompass the intricacies of diagnosis and medical care, the establishment of daily care routines, the crafting of a secure environment, and the navigation of the emotional and legal hurdles that caregivers often face. With the insights gleaned from this chapter, you will find yourself more adept at traversing the intricate landscape of vascular dementia, enabling you to offer both compassionate and effective care to your cherished one.

CHAPTER 3
DIAGNOSIS AND HEALTH CARE

The timely identification of the condition and the provision of appropriate medical attention are essential in the management of vascular dementia. This chapter delves into the intricacies of the diagnostic process, emphasizing the vital role of cultivating a robust relationship with healthcare providers to secure the finest care for your cherished one.

Identifying Initial Indicators

The progression of vascular dementia is often a slow and insidious journey, with early signs that may be faint and easily missed by those who encounter them. Yet, acknowledging these initial indicators is essential for prompt action. Among the early signs that one might observe are:

- Instances of memory lapses, especially those pertaining to short-term memory loss

- The struggle to maintain focus or engage in dialogue

- Wrestling with the intricacies of planning, the art of organization, and the challenges of problem-solving tasks

- Shifts in emotional state or character, manifesting as heightened irritability or a descent into melancholy

- A sudden onset of confusion, particularly in the aftermath of a stroke or transient ischemic attack (TIA), can be a disorienting experience.

Should you observe any of these symptoms in your cherished companion, it becomes imperative to pursue a medical evaluation without delay. Timely identification of the condition can significantly enhance management strategies, ultimately elevating the quality of life for both the individual and their caregiver.

The Process of Diagnosis

The journey to diagnose vascular dementia unfolds

through a series of meticulous steps, often necessitating the collaborative efforts of a diverse array of healthcare professionals, such as primary care physicians, neurologists, and neuropsychologists. In the diagnostic process, one may often encounter a variety of essential components:

- The healthcare provider shall meticulously gather a comprehensive medical history, delving into any prior strokes, transient ischemic attacks, or other conditions that could potentially influence the flow of blood to the brain. Inquiries will also be made regarding any familial history of dementia or cardiovascular concerns.

- A comprehensive physical examination shall be undertaken to evaluate the individual's overall health and to uncover any indications of neurological or cardiovascular issues. This may encompass the assessment of blood pressure, heart rate, and reflexes.

- In the realm of healthcare, the provider embarks on a meticulous journey through a series of neurological tests, each designed to unveil the intricacies of cognitive function, memory, language skills, coordination, and reflexes. These assessments serve to illuminate regions of the brain that might be impacted by vascular dementia.

- In the realm of cognitive and neuropsychological

testing, a variety of specialized assessments are employed to evaluate an individual's cognitive abilities. These tests delve into the intricacies of memory, attention, problem-solving, and language skills, revealing the depths of the mind's capabilities. These assessments unveil a comprehensive portrait of the individual's cognitive strengths and weaknesses, aiding in the distinction of vascular dementia from other forms of dementia.

- Imaging Studies: Techniques for brain imaging, including magnetic resonance imaging (MRI) and computed tomography (CT) scans, serve to unveil the intricate structure of the brain and identify any irregularities that may exist. The imaging studies unveil crucial evidence of strokes, TIAs, or small vessel disease, all of which stand as prevalent culprits behind vascular dementia.

- In the realm of medical exploration, blood tests may be undertaken to eliminate the possibility of other conditions that could evoke similar symptoms, including thyroid disorders, vitamin deficiencies, or infections. These assessments serve to guarantee a precise diagnosis and the right course of treatment.

Collaborating with Healthcare Professionals

Establishing a robust connection with healthcare providers is crucial for the effective management of vascular dementia. Consider these suggestions for collaborating with healthcare professionals to secure the finest care for your cherished one:

- Engage in transparent and sincere dialogue with your healthcare providers. Express any worries, insights, or alterations in your beloved's state, and pose inquiries to illuminate any ambiguities or uncertainties. Effective communication enables healthcare providers to grasp the unique needs of your loved one, allowing them to customize their care with precision.

- As a caregiver, you hold a vital position in championing the needs and desires of your loved one. Take the initiative to gather information, engage in conversations about treatment possibilities, and make certain that the desires of your loved one are honored. Advocacy serves as a vital force, ensuring that your cherished one is granted the utmost care and support they deserve.

- Collaboration: Foster collaboration among various healthcare providers to guarantee a thorough and unified approach to care. Maintain a meticulous record of appointments, medications, and treatment plans, ensuring that this vital information is communicated to all pertinent professionals. The orchestration of care serves to bridge the divides in treatment, fostering improved health outcomes along the way.

- Reach out to healthcare providers for assistance, ensuring that both your loved one and you receive the care and guidance needed. A multitude of healthcare professionals stand ready to offer invaluable resources, including support groups, counseling services, and educational materials, to assist you in navigating the intricate challenges of caregiving. The assistance offered by healthcare providers has the potential to ease the weight of stress and the burdens that often accompany the role of a caregiver.

- Regular follow-up appointments serve as a crucial means of tracking the progression of vascular dementia, allowing for timely adjustments to the treatment plan as circumstances evolve. Make it a priority to attend every scheduled appointment, remaining ever watchful for any shifts in your loved one's condition. A timely follow-up serves to guarantee that your cherished one continues to receive the care that is both ongoing and fitting.

Care and Oversight

Although a definitive cure for vascular dementia remains elusive, various treatment and management strategies exist that can ease symptoms and enhance the quality of life for those affected by this condition. Commonly employed methods in the treatment and management of vascular dementia include the following approaches:

- In the realm of healthcare, practitioners often turn to the prescription of medications as a means to alleviate various symptoms. These may include challenges related to memory, fluctuations in mood, and disturbances in sleep patterns. Moreover, the administration of medications aimed at managing underlying conditions—such as hypertension, diabetes, and elevated cholesterol levels—can significantly mitigate the risk of additional vascular harm.

- Transformative Choices: Embracing a healthier way of living can enhance one's overall well-being and diminish the likelihood of additional vascular harm. Inspire your cherished companion to partake in consistent physical activity, embrace a balanced diet, steer clear of smoking, and moderate their alcohol intake.

- Rehabilitation encompasses a range of therapies—occupational, physical, and speech—that serve to empower individuals grappling with vascular dementia.

Through these interventions, they can strive to uphold their independence while enhancing both cognitive and physical capabilities. Rehabilitation services offer focused interventions designed to tackle particular challenges and enhance overall well-being.

- Supportive therapies, including counseling, support groups, and social activities, serve as vital resources for individuals grappling with vascular dementia and their caregivers, aiding them in navigating the emotional and psychological challenges posed by the condition. The therapies foster a profound sense of community and support, alleviating the burdens of isolation and stress.

Through a deep comprehension of the diagnostic journey and a spirit of collaboration with healthcare professionals, caregivers can guarantee that their cherished ones receive the utmost care in the face of vascular dementia. In the ensuing chapters, we shall delve into pragmatic approaches for overseeing daily care, crafting a secure atmosphere, and navigating the emotional and legal dimensions of caregiving. With a wealth of knowledge and unwavering support, caregivers embark on a journey through the intricate landscape of vascular dementia, offering care that is both compassionate and profoundly effective.

CHAPTER 4
DAILY NURTURING AND SYMPTOM MANAGEMENT

To care for a cherished individual grappling with vascular dementia is to embark on a journey filled with a myriad of symptoms and daily trials. Creating structured routines, utilizing impactful communication methods, and addressing behavioral challenges can profoundly improve the well-being of both the individual and their caregiver. This chapter offers insightful guidance and strategies for the everyday nurturing and management of symptoms.

1. Creating a Routine

Establishing a well-organized and consistent daily routine serves to alleviate confusion and anxiety for those navigating the challenges of vascular dementia. Consistency weaves a tapestry of stability and security, guiding them through the intricacies of their day with greater ease. Consider these insights for crafting impactful routines:

- Consistency is key: Establish a routine for rising each morning, enjoying meals, engaging in activities, and retiring for the night. Consistency serves to strengthen memory and fosters a comforting sense of normalcy.

- To simplify, divide tasks into straightforward, manageable steps. Provide straightforward and succinct guidance, steering clear of inundating your dear one with intricate or numerous tasks simultaneously.

- Employ visual aids, including calendars, clocks, and labels, to strengthen the routine and serve as reminders. Labeling drawers and cabinets serves as a guiding beacon, allowing individuals to effortlessly locate their belongings with ease.

- Flexibility is key; although routines hold significance, it is equally vital to embrace adaptability in response to the evolving needs and preferences of your loved one. One must remain ready to modify the schedule as necessary, ensuring that their comfort and well-being are prioritized.

2. Strategies for Effective Communication

Mastering the art of communication is essential for grasping and addressing the needs of those affected by vascular dementia. Presented below are several strategies to elevate the art of communication:

- In the pursuit of understanding, one must articulate thoughts with deliberate slowness, ensuring each word resonates with clarity, while embracing the elegance of simplicity in language. Steer clear of intricate sentences and vague ideas. Do not hesitate to reiterate details when needed, and maintain a sense of patience.

- Nonverbal Communication: Observe the subtle nuances of nonverbal cues, including the delicate play of facial expressions, the eloquence of gestures, and the silent language of body posture. Such observations can unveil profound understandings of your cherished one's feelings and desires.

- Engage in the art of active listening by ensuring your gaze meets that of the speaker, offering gentle nods of understanding, and interjecting with verbal affirmations that convey your attentiveness. Allow your beloved the grace of time to formulate their thoughts, refraining from interjecting or completing their sentences.

- Inspire your cherished one to find their voice, even when the path of communication proves to be difficult. Affirm their emotions and offer comfort, highlighting the significance of their thoughts and feelings.

3. Addressing Behavioral Symptoms

In individuals grappling with vascular dementia, behavioral symptoms frequently emerge, presenting a formidable challenge for those tasked with their care. Grasping the fundamental reasons and utilizing potent approaches can aid in tackling these behaviors:

- Recognizing Triggers: Carefully observe and record behaviors to unveil patterns and discern potential triggers. Gaining insight into the triggers of specific behaviors can empower you to establish proactive strategies.

- Redirection: In moments when your cherished companion displays difficult behaviors, softly guide their focus toward an alternative activity or subject. Involving them in a cherished pastime or soothing endeavor can serve to ease the tension of the moment.

- Craft a serene and tranquil atmosphere to alleviate restlessness and unease.

Reduce noise, eliminate clutter, and remove distractions, while ensuring that the living space is bright and inviting.

- Employ the power of positive reinforcement to nurture and promote the behaviors you wish to see flourish. Celebrate and acknowledge your beloved's achievements, regardless of their size.

4. Self-Care and Cleanliness

Providing support with personal care and hygiene stands as a fundamental element of the caregiving journey. Upholding cleanliness and grooming serves to elevate the comfort and dignity of your cherished companion. Here are a few suggestions for delivering personal care:

- Approach personal care tasks with a profound sense of sensitivity and respect, honoring the dignity of each individual involved. Elucidate each stage of the journey and invite your cherished companion to share their thoughts and collaborate.

- It is essential to guarantee that the bathroom and other spaces designated for personal care are both secure and easily accessible. Incorporate grab bars, non-slip mats, and various safety features to safeguard against potential accidents.

- Establish a consistent routine for bathing,

grooming, and dressing. Establishing a sense of consistency may foster a greater sense of comfort in your loved one, reducing their resistance to these tasks.

- Embrace the use of gentle, soothing products and techniques to elevate the experience of comfort. Observe closely the inclinations of your cherished ones, as well as any subtle indications of unease or annoyance that may arise.

5. Nutrition and Hydration

The significance of proper nutrition and hydration cannot be overstated, as they play a vital role in the overall health and well-being of those grappling with vascular dementia. In the capacity of a caregiver, you hold a crucial responsibility in safeguarding the well-being of your loved one, ensuring they enjoy a balanced diet and remain adequately hydrated. Within these pages lie a collection of strategies designed to champion the cause of good nutrition and hydration:

- A balanced diet encompasses a rich tapestry of nutritious foods drawn from every food group. It invites an array of fruits, vibrant vegetables, wholesome grains, lean proteins, and dairy, each contributing to the symphony of health and vitality. Steer clear of processed foods and limit your intake of excessive sugars.

- Petite repasts: Present a series of smaller, more frequent meals and snacks to grace the day. This approach can gracefully adapt to fluctuations in appetite, thereby mitigating the potential for both overeating and under eating.

- Hydration: Foster a routine of fluid consumption by providing water, herbal teas, and an array of other non-caffeinated drinks. Be vigilant for indications of dehydration, including a parched mouth, deep-hued urine, and an overwhelming sense of fatigue.

- Support may be offered during mealtime, should it be required. Utilize adaptive utensils and plate guards to empower your loved one in their journey toward greater independence during mealtime. Foster a serene and inviting atmosphere during meals, transforming the experience into one of delight.

6. Captivating Pursuits

Involving your cherished companion in purposeful pursuits can elevate their mental acuity, enrich their emotional health, and improve their overall existence. Herein lie a collection of pursuits that promise to be both delightful and advantageous:

- Engage in pursuits that awaken the intellect, embracing the challenge of puzzles, the joy of reading, the intrigue of memory games, and the creativity found in arts and crafts.

Engaging in these pursuits can nurture cognitive faculties and foster a profound sense of achievement.

- Encourage the embrace of regular physical activity, encompassing the simple joys of walking, the soothing motions of stretching, and the gentle rhythm of light exercises. Engaging in physical activity holds the promise of bolstering cardiovascular health, alleviating stress, and uplifting one's mood.

- Encourage the blossoming of social bonds by inviting your cherished one to partake in group activities, family gatherings, and community events. Engaging in social interaction has the power to alleviate the burdens of isolation and offer a comforting embrace of emotional support.

- Encourage your beloved to delve into the pursuits that ignite their passion, be it the nurturing of a garden, the art of cooking, the melodies of music, or the strokes of a paintbrush. Participating in beloved and pleasurable pursuits can elevate one's spirits and instill a profound sense of purpose.

Through the application of these pragmatic approaches to daily care and symptom management, caregivers have the opportunity to cultivate a supportive and nurturing atmosphere for their cherished ones grappling with vascular dementia. In the forthcoming chapters, we shall delve into the art of crafting a secure and nurturing atmosphere, examining the intricacies of emotional and mental wellness, while also traversing the landscape of legal and financial matters. With a blend of wisdom and heartfelt compassion, caregivers possess the remarkable ability to transform the lives of those entrusted to their care.

CHAPTER 5
CRAFTING A SANCTUARY OF SAFETY AND SUPPORT

Creating a safe and nurturing environment is vital for the well-being and quality of life of those living with vascular dementia. An environment thoughtfully designed can significantly lower the likelihood of mishaps, alleviate disorientation, and foster a sense of autonomy. This chapter offers insightful guidance on enhancing home safety through thoughtful modifications, the use of adaptive equipment, and the creation of a community that embraces the needs of those living with dementia.

1. Enhancements for Home Safety

Transforming the home environment to cater to the unique needs of those living with vascular dementia can profoundly improve their safety and comfort. Consider these essential aspects when embarking on the journey of enhancing home safety modifications:

- Illumination: It is essential to guarantee that every corner of the home is adequately illuminated, thereby minimizing the potential for falls and mishaps. In the quiet hours of the night, let gentle nightlights illuminate the hallways, bathrooms, and bedrooms, offering a soft glow that guides the way and ensures safety in the darkness. One might contemplate the installation of motion-sensor lights, enhancing both convenience and safety in one's surroundings.

- In the realm of flooring, it is essential to eliminate any loose rugs, clutter, and obstacles that may pose a risk of tripping or falling. In the realms of bathrooms and kitchens, it is wise to employ non-slip mats, while also ensuring that the flooring remains even and well-maintained.

- In the realm of interior design, one must

thoughtfully arrange the furniture to forge clear pathways, ensuring that the space remains uncluttered and inviting. It is essential to guarantee that chairs and sofas possess a robust construction and are set at a suitable height, facilitating the ease of both sitting and standing. Steer clear of furniture adorned with sharp edges, or consider employing corner protectors to safeguard against potential injuries.

- In the realm of bathroom safety, one must consider the installation of grab bars and handrails, especially in proximity to the toilet and shower, ensuring a secure environment for all who enter. Employ a shower chair or bench alongside a handheld showerhead to enhance the safety and comfort of your bathing experience. It may be wise to contemplate the installation of a raised toilet seat, alongside the addition of non-slip mats within the shower and bathtub.

- In the realm of culinary endeavors, it is paramount to prioritize safety. One should ensure that commonly utilized items are conveniently positioned within arm's reach, thereby eliminating the necessity for precarious climbing or stretching. Employ devices equipped with automatic shut-off capabilities and eliminate or deactivate those appliances that may present a hazard. Ensure that sharp objects, cleaning supplies, and medications are stored securely and kept out of reach.

- Doors and windows stand as the guardians of our sanctuaries; it is imperative to ensure they are fortified with secure locks that offer both safety and ease of use. One might contemplate the installation of childproof locks or alarms, a prudent measure to deter any unintended wandering. Employ decals or striking colors on glass doors and expansive windows to avert mishaps.

- In the realm of emergency preparedness, it is essential to devise a comprehensive plan, ensuring that every family member and caregiver is well-acquainted with its details. Ensure that emergency contact information is easily accessible, and contemplate the use of a medical alert system for an extra layer of security.

2. Innovative Tools and Technologies for Adaptation

Adaptive equipment and technologies serve as vital tools for individuals grappling with vascular dementia, empowering them to uphold their independence and enhance their quality of life. Presented here are a selection of valuable tools and devices worthy of your consideration:

- Mobility aids, including canes, walkers, and wheelchairs, serve as essential companions in the journey of safe movement, helping to prevent falls and ensuring a steadier path forward. It is essential to guarantee that these aids are fitted with precision and maintained on a regular basis.

- Communication Devices: One might contemplate the utilization of various communication devices, including picture boards, voice-activated assistants, or specialized applications, to enhance the flow of communication and offer reminders for daily undertakings.

- Memory aids serve as invaluable companions in the journey of daily life. Tools such as calendars, clocks, and electronic reminders assist individuals in navigating the complexities of appointments, medications, and the myriad of daily activities that demand attention. Digital photo frames, showcasing beloved faces and cherished places, offer a sense of solace and help to alleviate disorientation.

- In the realm of safeguarding, one might consider the installation of monitoring systems—devices like motion sensors, door alarms, and video cameras. These tools not only enhance safety but also offer a reassuring sense of tranquility for those entrusted with care. These systems possess the capability to observe activity and deter wandering.

- Employing assistive devices, including reachers, grabbers, and adaptive utensils, can transform daily tasks into endeavors that are not only easier but also more manageable. These devices serve as invaluable companions, empowering individuals to uphold their independence and engage in the essential activities of daily living.

3. Creating a Community Embracing Dementia Awareness

To cultivate a community that embraces those affected by dementia, one must embark on a journey of awareness, nurture a deep understanding, and extend unwavering support to both individuals living with dementia and their dedicated caregivers. Here are several approaches to cultivate a nurturing and inclusive community:

- Enlightenment and Understanding: Illuminate the minds of family, friends, neighbors, and community members regarding the nuances of vascular dementia and the profound effects it can have. Detail the ways to identify symptoms, extend support, and engage in meaningful communication with those living with dementia.

- Support Groups: Consider joining or creating support groups for those living with dementia and their caregivers. Within these groups, individuals find a sanctuary where they can share their experiences, exchange valuable advice, and extend emotional support to one another.

- In the realm of community support, one may find solace in the offerings of adult day care centers, respite care services, and programs designed with the needs of those facing dementia in mind. These resources offer invaluable support and open doors to opportunities for social engagement.

- Champion the cause of policies and initiatives that uplift individuals living with dementia and their devoted caregivers. Collaborate with community organizations, healthcare professionals, and governmental bodies to enhance awareness and facilitate access to essential services.

- Fostering Inclusivity: Inspire community

organizations to provide activities and events that are friendly to those living with dementia. Among these offerings are memory cafes, art classes, music therapy sessions, and exercise programs, all thoughtfully crafted to meet the unique needs of individuals living with dementia.

Through the careful implementation of home safety modifications, the use of adaptive equipment, and the fostering of community-building strategies, caregivers have the opportunity to cultivate a safe and nurturing environment for their cherished ones living with vascular dementia. In the ensuing chapters, we shall embark on a journey to delve into the intricacies of emotional and mental well-being, traverse the landscape of legal and financial considerations, and meticulously plan for advanced care. With a blend of understanding and heartfelt attention, caregivers possess the remarkable ability to transform the lives of those entrusted to their care.

CHAPTER 6
EMOTIONAL AND MENTAL HEALTH

The emotional and mental health of both the caregiver and the individual living with vascular dementia stands as a pivotal element in the caregiving journey. Providing care for a cherished individual grappling with dementia can weigh heavily on the heart, often giving rise to a tumult of emotions such as stress, anxiety, and despair. This chapter delves into the various strategies one can employ to navigate the emotional landscape of caregiving, offering insights into stress management techniques and the importance of seeking support through counseling and community groups.

Navigating the Emotional Landscape

To care for an individual grappling with vascular dementia is to navigate a complex tapestry of emotions, weaving together threads of love and fulfillment alongside those of frustration and grief. It is crucial to acknowledge and confront these emotions, as doing so plays a vital role in preserving one's mental well-being and ensuring the delivery of compassionate care. Within the realm of caregiving, one may discover various strategies to navigate the emotional landscape that accompanies this profound responsibility:

- Recognize Your Emotions: It is essential to recognize and embrace your emotions, regardless of what they might entail. It is entirely natural to navigate through a tapestry of emotions, weaving together threads of sadness, anger, guilt, and joy. Embrace these emotions, permitting yourself to experience them free from any judgment.

- Articulate Your Feelings: Seek out constructive avenues to convey your emotions, whether it be through heartfelt conversations with a trusted confidant or family member, penning your thoughts in a journal, or immersing yourself in creative pursuits like painting or music. Articulating your emotions can offer solace and aid in the navigation of your inner landscape.

- Consider Reaching Out for Guidance: Should you struggle to navigate your emotions, it may be wise to seek the support of a mental health professional. Engaging in therapy or counseling offers a sanctuary where one can delve into their emotions and cultivate effective coping mechanisms. A therapist can guide you through the intricate journey of caregiving, offering solace and understanding in times of difficulty.

Methods for Managing Stress

The journey of caregiving often unfolds under a veil of stress, a relentless companion that can cast shadows upon both physical and mental well-being. Employing stress management techniques can enhance your wellbeing and enable you to offer improved care for your cherished one. Within the realm of stress management, several strategies emerge as particularly effective:

- Engaging in the practices of mindfulness and meditation serves as a balm for the weary soul, offering a pathway to diminish stress and cultivate a profound sense of relaxation. Mindfulness is the art of immersing oneself in the present moment, embracing it with an open heart and a non-judgmental spirit. Through the practice of meditation, one may find solace for the restless mind, fostering a greater capacity to navigate the tumultuous waters of stress.

- Engaging in regular physical activity serves as a formidable antidote to the burdens of stress. Engaging in exercise unleashes a cascade of endorphins, those delightful chemicals that elevate one's spirits and alleviate the burdens of stress. Seek out pursuits that bring you joy, be it a leisurely walk, the grace of yoga, or the rhythm of dance, and weave them into the fabric of your everyday life.

- Engaging in deep breathing exercises serves as a powerful antidote to stress, fostering a sense of tranquility and relaxation. Engage in the art of deep breathing by drawing in air gently through your nose, pausing for a moment to hold that breath, and then releasing it slowly through your mouth. Engage in this practice multiple times to soothe both your mind and body.

- Mastering the art of time management can significantly alleviate stress, as it empowers one to prioritize tasks and carve out moments for self-care. Devise a daily itinerary that thoughtfully incorporates moments for caregiving duties, professional obligations, and personal leisure pursuits. Assign responsibilities when feasible and steer clear of taking on more than you can handle.

Discovering avenues for support and guidance

Reaching out to those who comprehend the trials of caregiving can offer profound emotional and practical support. Support groups and counseling serve as a beacon of community, alleviating the weight of isolation while imparting valuable coping strategies. Here are several avenues to seek assistance:

- Consider becoming a part of a caregiver support group, whether in your local community or through online platforms. Within these groups, individuals find a sanctuary where they can openly share their experiences, seek guidance, and draw upon the emotional support of those who traverse similar paths. Support groups possess the remarkable ability to provide profound insights and cultivate a deep sense of connection among individuals.

- Numerous organizations provide invaluable resources and support for those who care for individuals living with dementia. These organizations have the potential to offer a wealth of educational materials, host enlightening workshops, and facilitate supportive groups for those in need. Among the notable examples are the Alzheimer's Association,

Dementia Friends, and various local advocacy groups dedicated to dementia.

- Engaging in counseling or therapy, whether on an individual basis or within a group setting, may prove beneficial in navigating the emotional complexities that accompany the role of a caregiver. A licensed therapist possesses the expertise to guide you in cultivating coping strategies, enhancing your communication skills, and skillfully navigating the complexities of difficult emotions. In the realm of personal growth, therapy emerges as a sanctuary, offering a secure and private environment where one can delve into their emotions and seek the wisdom of guidance.

- Respite care serves as a beacon of temporary relief for caregivers, granting them a much-needed pause by providing short-term care for their cherished ones. This grants you the opportunity to pause and center your attention on your own wellbeing. Respite care may be offered by skilled caregivers, adult day care facilities, or specialized respite care programs. Regularly stepping away can serve as a safeguard against burnout, enhancing your capacity to offer care effectively.

- Discover the wealth of community resources available to provide invaluable support for caregivers. Numerous communities offer a variety of programs and services aimed at supporting caregivers, including training opportunities, counseling services, and engaging social activities. These resources offer tangible support and avenues for social interaction.

Fostering Emotional Resilience

Fostering emotional resilience serves as a guiding light through the trials of caregiving, allowing one to uphold their mental wellbeing amidst the storm. Within these pages lie a collection of strategies designed to cultivate resilience:

- Embrace the art of positive thinking by nurturing a mindset that highlights the strengths and uplifting facets of caregiving. Embrace gratitude by recognizing the small triumphs and fleeting moments of joy that grace your path as a caregiver. Embracing a mindset of positivity has the power to transform your perspective and enhance your overall outlook on life.

- Embrace the art of self-compassion by extending to yourself the warmth of kindness and the embrace of understanding. Understand that the journey of caregiving is fraught with challenges, and it is perfectly acceptable to experience tough days. Refrain from harsh judgments upon yourself and take a moment to acknowledge that you are striving to give your utmost.

- Establishing healthy boundaries is essential for safeguarding your mental and emotional wellbeing. Establish boundaries around your caregiving duties and carve out moments for pursuits that ignite your joy and foster relaxation. Articulate your needs and establish your boundaries with your family, inviting their support in the journey ahead.

- Embrace the power of supportive relationships, those that envelop you in encouragement, understanding, and empathy. Connect with friends, family, and support groups to seek the comfort of emotional support. Establishing a robust support network can alleviate feelings of isolation and foster a deeper sense of connection.

In attending to the emotional and mental wellbeing of both

the caregiver and the individual navigating the challenges of vascular dementia, one can cultivate a more supportive and nurturing atmosphere. In the chapters that follow, we shall delve into the intricate realms of legal and financial considerations, the nuances of advanced care planning, and the various resources and support networks available to us. With a blend of understanding and heartfelt attention, caregivers possess the remarkable ability to transform the lives of those entrusted to their care.

CHAPTER 7

CONSIDERATIONS OF LEGAL AND FINANCIAL NATURE

The journey through the intricate legal and financial realms of caregiving often presents itself as a formidable challenge. Thorough planning and a clear comprehension of one's legal rights and responsibilities stand as vital pillars in safeguarding the well-being and protection of both the caregiver and the individual grappling with vascular dementia. This chapter unveils crucial insights into the realm of legal rights, the art of future planning, and the pathways to securing financial assistance.

Comprehending One's Legal Entitlements

Grasping the intricacies of your legal rights as a caregiver, alongside the rights of the individual grappling with vascular dementia, is of paramount importance. Within the realm of legal considerations, several pivotal aspects demand attention:

Authority to Act on Behalf: A power of attorney (POA) serves as a legal instrument, bestowing upon a chosen individual the capacity to make decisions in the stead of another person. Two primary forms of Power of Attorney hold significance in the realm of caregiving:

- A Medical Power of Attorney grants the appointed individual the authority to make healthcare decisions for the person afflicted with dementia, should they find themselves unable to do so.

- A Financial Power of Attorney bestows the authority to oversee financial matters, encompassing the payment of bills, the management of bank accounts, and the handling of investments.

Advance Directives: These are legal documents that articulate an individual's desires regarding medical care, should they find themselves unable to convey their wishes. Among the various forms of advance directives, several stand out:

- A Living Will is a document that delineates the medical treatments and life-sustaining measures an individual desires or wishes to forgo in specific circumstances.

- A Do Not Resuscitate (DNR) Order signifies the individual's wish to forgo cardiopulmonary resuscitation (CPR) in the event that their heart ceases to beat or they stop breathing altogether.

In instances where a person afflicted with dementia finds

themselves unable to make decisions independently and has not appointed a Power of Attorney, the court may intervene to appoint a guardian or conservator, thereby entrusting them with the responsibility of making decisions on the individual's behalf. Guardianship generally encompasses decisions related to personal and healthcare matters, whereas conservatorship pertains to financial affairs.

Individuals grappling with dementia are entitled to receive

the medical care that is fitting for their condition, to be treated with the utmost dignity and respect, and to have their privacy safeguarded. It is essential for caregivers to remain cognizant of these rights and to champion the needs of their loved ones whenever the situation demands it.

Envisioning Tomorrow

Envisioning the future is crucial to guarantee that the requirements of both the caregiver and the individual living with dementia are fulfilled.

Here are a few steps to contemplate:

- Legal Documentation: It is imperative to ensure that all essential legal documents, including Powers of Attorney, advance directives, wills, and trusts, are meticulously completed and kept current. Seek the guidance of an attorney well-versed in elder law or estate planning to guarantee that all legal matters are meticulously attended to.

- In the realm of financial foresight, it is prudent to engage with a financial advisor who can assist in crafting a thorough financial strategy. This plan should meticulously consider the various expenses associated with caregiving, medical needs, and the intricacies of long-term care. Explore possibilities like long-term care insurance, annuities, and various financial instruments that may assist in managing the expenses associated with care.

- Medicaid and Medicare: Delve into the intricacies of eligibility requirements and the array of benefits offered by Medicaid and Medicare, both of which serve to alleviate the financial burdens associated with medical care and long-term care. Medicaid extends its protective embrace to those with limited financial means, ensuring health coverage for low-income individuals. In contrast, Medicare stands as a federal bastion of health insurance, dedicated to serving those aged 65 and above, as well as individuals grappling with specific disabilities.

- Long-Term Care: Delve into the various avenues available for long-term care, including in-home assistance, adult day care centers, assisted living facilities, and nursing homes. Evaluate the expenses, accessibility, and standard of care offered by these alternatives to ascertain the most suitable choice for your cherished one's requirements.

Charting the Course of Financial Aid

Securing financial assistance can ease the weight of the financial responsibilities that come with caregiving. Within the realm of financial support, several avenues beckon for consideration:

In the realm of caregiving, a tapestry of government programs unfolds, offering both financial assistance and unwavering support to those who tend to individuals grappling with dementia. Illustrations encompass:

- Social Security Disability Insurance (SSDI) offers financial assistance to those who find themselves unable to engage in work due to a disability, such as dementia.

- Supplemental Security Income (SSI) provides

financial support to individuals who are low-income and fall into the categories of aged, blind, or disabled.

- The Department of Veterans Affairs (VA) extends a range of benefits and services to veterans grappling with dementia and their caregivers. These provisions encompass healthcare, disability compensation, and pension benefits, all designed to support those who have served.

- In the realm of community resources, one may discover a wealth of local and national organizations poised to provide financial assistance, grants, and invaluable support services for caregivers and those navigating the challenges of dementia. Among the notable examples are the Alzheimer's Association, Area Agencies on Aging, and various local advocacy groups dedicated to dementia.

- Numerous nonprofit organizations extend their hands to offer financial assistance, respite care, and a variety of support services tailored for caregivers. Investigate and connect with organizations that provide resources and support for those caring for individuals with dementia.

- Employer Benefits: A number of employers extend their support to caregivers through various benefits, including flexible work schedules, paid family leave, and employee assistance programs. Inquire with your employer regarding the benefits that may be accessible to you.

Through a deep comprehension of your legal rights, thoughtful planning for the future, and the pursuit of financial assistance, you can create a foundation of support and protection for both yourself and your cherished ones. In the forthcoming chapters, we shall delve into the intricacies of advanced care planning, alongside the resources and support networks that accompany it. With a blend of understanding and heartfelt attention, caregivers possess the remarkable ability to transform the lives of those entrusted to their care.

CHAPTER 8

PLANNING AHEAD FOR CARE

It's more and more important to plan for advanced care as vascular dementia gets worse. This part talks about hospice and palliative care, decisions about end-of-life care, and how to help the caregiver get through the grieving process. It is important to be ready for these situations so that you can honor your loved one's wishes and be ready for the mental challenges that may come up.

Decisions about end-of-life care

Making choices about end-of-life care is very personal and can be hard to do. But talking about and writing down these choices early on can help both the helper and the person with dementia understand them better and feel better. Here are some important things to think about when planning end-of-life care:

- Advance Directives: Make sure that any living wills or DNR orders that you have are filled out and up to date. These papers spell out your loved one's wishes for medical care and steps to keep them alive in case they become unable to say what they want.

- Comfort care: Make sure your loved one is comfortable and keeps their respect. This could mean taking care of pain and other symptoms, making sure the setting is calm and soothing, and giving emotional support.

- Medical Interventions: Talk to your loved one about what they want when it comes to medical interventions like food tubes, ventilators, and CPR. In tough situations, knowing what they want can help you make decisions.

- Quality of Life: Put your loved one's physical, mental, and spiritual needs first when you think about their quality of life. This could mean doing things that are important to you, spending time with people you care about, and looking for spiritual or religious support.

Hospice and end-of-life care

Hospice care and palliative care are specialized services that help people with major illnesses and their families. Instead of treating illnesses, these services focus on making people's lives better and making them feel better. Knowing the differences between hospice care and palliative care can help you make better choices about how to care for your loved one:

- Palliative Care: This type of care can be given at any stage of a serious sickness and along with treatments that are meant to cure the illness. Its main goals are to control symptoms, offer mental support, and raise quality of life. A group of health care professionals, such as doctors, nurses, social workers, and pastors, often provide palliative care.

- Usually lacking more than six months to live, hospice care is a kind of palliative treatment administered to someone approaching the end of their life. Rather of aiming at a cure for the illness, hospice care emphasizes comfort and support. A hospital, a hospice, or the patient's own house can all be the venue for hospice care. Managing discomfort, providing mental support, and helping with everyday chores comprise hospice care.

- Advantages of Hospice and Palliative Care: For those

with dementia and their caregivers, both palliative care and hospice can be quite beneficial. These services provide all kinds of help, like medical care, mental and spiritual support, and help with everyday tasks. Hospice and palliative care can make it easier on caregivers and make sure that your loved one gets caring, respectful care.

Getting the caregiver through grief and loss

Being a caregiver for a loved one with vascular dementia means going through grief and loss as well as the physical and mental demands of caregiving. It is very important to help parents through this process for their own health. These are some ways to deal with loss and grief:

- Anticipatory Grief: Anticipatory grief is the mental pain that comes from knowing that a loved one is getting worse or dying. Know that it's okay to feel sad before the real loss happens. Let yourself cry, and get help from family, friends, or a therapist.

- Self-Compassion: Show yourself compassion by being kind and understanding to yourself. Realize that both caring for someone and grieving are hard, and that it's okay to feel a lot of different feelings. Let yourself cry and take time to care for yourself.

- Looking for Help: Check out support groups, counseling services, and other resources in your neighborhood. Talking about your thoughts and feelings with people who understand can help you feel better and less alone. Support groups can help you learn new things and find ways to deal with problems.

- Rituals and Memorials: To honor the life and memory of your loved one, make rituals or memorials. This could mean having a funeral service, making a memory book, planting a tree, or doing things that your loved one liked. Memorials and rituals can help you deal with your loss and give you a sense of closure.

- Professional Help: You might want to talk to a loss counselor or therapist for professional help. They can give you expert help and support as you go through the grieving process. Therapy can help you figure out how to deal with your feelings, explore them, and find a way to heal.

- Keeping in Touch: Keep in touch with family, friends, and support networks. Making friends can help you feel like you belong, give you mental support, and help you with everyday tasks. When things get tough, lean on your support network and let other people help you.

Caregivers can make sure that their loved ones get kind and

respectful care by planning ahead for advanced care and dealing with the emotional parts of sadness and loss. In the last chapter, we'll talk about the tools and support networks that caregivers can use. Caregivers can make a difference in the lives of the people they care for by learning about them and treating them with kindness.

CONCLUSION

Caring for a loved one who has vascular dementia is a journey full of unique difficulties, deep feelings, and times when you feel very connected to that person. The goal of "Vascular Dementia: A Caregiver's Handbook" is to give you the information, tools, and support you need to walk this path with kindness and confidence. This handbook covers all aspects of caregiving, from knowing the medical side of vascular dementia to managing daily care, making sure the environment is safe, taking care of the person's emotional health, and making plans for long-term care.

You are very important to the health and happiness of your loved one as a helper. Your love, commitment, and strength are what make the care you give possible. Remember to put your own health and happiness first, get help, and believe in your own power. You can make a change in the lives of the people you care about by giving yourself knowledge and tools.

Thanks for coming along with us on this trip. We hope that this guidebook is helpful and makes you feel better as you continue to care for your loved one with vascular dementia in a kind and effective way. You are not alone on this trip because people understand, help, and care about you. We can make a big difference in the lives of people with vascular dementia if we all work together.

Printed in Great Britain
by Amazon